The Type 2 Diabetes Solution:

Practical Strategies for a Healthier Life

By

John Poe

Table Of Contents

Introduction

Readers are welcomed into the world of diabetes care in the opening of "The Type 2 Diabetes Solution: Practical Strategies for a Healthier Life," which lays the groundwork for comprehending and tackling the difficulties of type 2 diabetes. The purpose of this part is to give readers a basic grasp of the illness and the vital role that lifestyle management plays in both prevention and control.

What Type 2 Diabetes Is

Insulin resistance and reduced insulin secretion are the main causes of type 2 diabetes, a chronic metabolic disease marked by high blood glucose levels.

Unlike type 1 diabetes, which is an autoimmune disease in which the immune system of the patient assaults the pancreatic cells that produce insulin, type 2 diabetes usually develops gradually over time and is frequently linked to lifestyle factors including obesity, poor food, and physical inactivity.

When a person has type 2 diabetes, their body develops resistance to the hormone insulin, which is released by the pancreas and aids in controlling blood sugar levels. Consequently, glucose accumulates in the bloodstream rather than being taken up by cells for energy, resulting in elevated blood sugar levels, which is a defining characteristic of diabetes. Long-term hyperglycemia raises the risk of major health issues such as heart disease, stroke, kidney disease, and nerve damage by causing damage to blood vessels and organs.

The Value of Responsible Lifestyle Management

Type 2 diabetes is influenced by both genetics and lifestyle choices, but lifestyle choices have a greater impact on the disease's incidence and progression. Studies have indicated that implementing health-conscious lifestyle practices can greatly lower the chance of acquiring type 2 diabetes and enhance the prognosis of individuals with the illness.

The cornerstone of diabetes treatment is lifestyle management, which includes a range of tactics like dietary adjustments, consistent exercise, managing weight, reducing stress, and quitting smoking. Individuals with type 2 diabetes can improve their general quality of life, avoid or delay problems, and better control their blood sugar levels by adopting positive adjustments in these areas.

We examine doable tactics and research-backed suggestions for adopting healthy lifestyle practices into day-to-day living in "The Type 2 Diabetes Solution." This book gives readers the knowledge and resources they need to take charge of their health and successfully manage type 2 diabetes, from meal planning and exercise regimens to stress management strategies and self-care routines.

Chapter One

An understanding of diabetes type two

We go deeper into the mechanics and variables of type 2 diabetes in this portion of "The Type 2 Diabetes Solution," giving readers a thorough grasp of the illness.

Factors at Risk and Their Causes

A complex interplay of genetic, environmental, and lifestyle variables contributes to type 2 diabetes. Diabetes is largely hereditary, but lifestyle factors including smoking, obesity, poor food, and physical inactivity can greatly raise an individual's risk of getting the disease. Age, race (African American,

Hispanic/Latino, Native American), gestational diabetes, polycystic ovarian syndrome (PCOS), family history of diabetes, and specific medical disorders (hypertension, dyslipidemia) are additional risk factors.

Signs and the Prognosis

Type 2 diabetes can develop gradually, and many people may not show any symptoms at first. Increased thirst, frequent urination, unexplained weight loss, exhaustion, hazy eyesight, sluggish wound healing, and recurring infections are typical signs of diabetes. On the other hand, some individuals could not show any symptoms at all or just have minor ones that go unnoticed for years. Blood tests that evaluate hemoglobin A1c (HbA1c) levels, oral glucose tolerance, or fasting blood glucose levels are commonly used to diagnose type 2 diabetes. When blood glucose levels are regularly higher than normal ranges, a diagnosis is verified.

Diabetes-Related Complications

Unmanaged or inadequately controlled type 2 diabetes can result in a variety of acute and chronic problems that impact different body organs and systems. While chronic complications can develop over time and include cardiovascular disease, neuropathy (nerve damage), nephropathy (kidney damage), retinopathy (eye damage), foot ulcers, and amputations, acute complications can include hyperglycemia (high blood sugar), which can lead to diabetic ketoacidosis

(DKA) or hyperosmolar hyperglycemic state (HHS).

For early detection, efficient care, and the avoidance of long-term consequences, it is crucial to comprehend the causes, symptoms, and possible complications associated with type 2 diabetes. Through educating readers about these facets of the disease and increasing awareness of it, "The Type 2 Diabetes Solution" enables readers to take charge of their health and well-being.

Chapter Two

Lifestyle Changes for the Management of Diabetes

We stress in "The Type 2 Diabetes Solution" how important lifestyle changes are to successfully control type 2 diabetes. Healthy lifestyle choices in terms of nutrition, exercise, and stress reduction can have a big impact on blood sugar regulation, lower the risk of complications, and enhance the general quality of life for people with diabetes.

Nutrition and Diet

Healthy, well-balanced diet is essential for managing diabetes. Important dietary guidelines consist of:

Carbohydrate Management: To avoid blood sugar spikes, choose complex carbs with a low glycemic index and keep an eye on your intake.

Portion control is the process of regulating serving sizes to avoid overindulging and control caloric intake.

Healthy Fats: Including foods high in heart-healthy fats, including nuts, seeds, avocados, and fatty fish, will help satiate hunger and maintain heart health.

Lean Proteins: Consuming lean protein sources to assist preserve muscle mass and control blood sugar levels, such as fish, poultry, tofu, and lentils.

Fruits and Vegetables: For optimum nutrition and blood sugar regulation, give priority to a range of vibrant fruits and vegetables that are high in vitamins, minerals, and fiber.

Physical Activity and Exercise

Frequent exercise is crucial for managing diabetes because it lowers blood sugar, increases insulin sensitivity, and lowers the risk of cardiovascular problems. Among the suggested workout guidelines are:

Aerobic exercise is defined as 150 minutes or more a week of moderate-intensity physical activity, such as brisk walking, cycling, swimming, or dancing.

Strength Training: Include workouts with resistance bands, free weights, or your body weight to increase muscle growth and enhance your metabolism in general.

Stretching and balancing exercises can improve flexibility and mobility while lowering the chance of falling.

Techniques for Relaxation and Stress Reduction

Prolonged stress can raise blood sugar and have a detrimental effect on managing diabetes. Better blood sugar control and emotional well-being can be achieved by incorporating relaxation and stress-reduction methods. Techniques for managing stress that work well include:

Mindfulness & Meditation: To lower tension and encourage relaxation, try mindfulness meditation, progressive muscle relaxation, or deep breathing techniques.

Yoga and Tai Chi: Engaging in mind-body exercises to enhance flexibility, balance, and mental clarity, such as yoga or tai chi.

Hobbies and Recreational Activities: Taking part in fun recreational activities, hobbies, or time spent in nature as a way to relax and rejuvenate. Type 2 diabetics can improve their general health, lower their reliance on medication, and successfully manage their disease over the long term by incorporating these lifestyle changes into their daily routines. "The Type 2 Diabetes Solution" offers helpful advice and methods for putting these lifestyle adjustments into practice.

Chapter Three

Options for Medication and Treatment

Even while changing one's lifestyle is essential for controlling type 2 diabetes,

medication and other treatment options are frequently required to attain ideal blood sugar control and avoid complications. We examine the several pharmacological therapies and therapy methods that are available for people with type 2 diabetes in "The Type 2 Diabetes Solution."
An Overview of Oral Drugs

Metformin: For type 2 diabetes, metformin is typically the first-line treatment. It functions by lowering the liver's synthesis of glucose, enhancing insulin sensitivity, and lowering the intestinal absorption of sugar.

Sulfonylureas: Sulfonylureas assist reduce blood sugar levels by stimulating the pancreas to release more insulin.

Glipizide, glyburide, and glimepiride are a few examples.

DPP-4 Inhibitors: By raising insulin secretion and lowering glucagon synthesis, dipeptidyl peptidase-4 (DPP-4) inhibitors contribute to blood sugar reduction. Saxagliptin, linagliptin, and sitagliptin are a few examples.

SGLT-2 Blockers: SGLT-2 inhibitors function by blocking the kidneys' ability to reabsorb glucose, which increases the amount of glucose excreted in the urine. Dapagliflozin, canagliflozin, and empagliflozin are a few examples.

Agonists of GLP-1 Receptors: Glucagon-like peptide-1 (GLP-1) receptor agonists reduce stomach emptying, increase satiety, inhibit glucagon secretion, and enhance insulin secretion. Liraglutide, exenatide, and dulaglutide are a few examples.

Insulin Treatment

Insulin therapy may be required for type 2 diabetics whose blood sugar control is inadequate when treated with oral medicines alone. The goal of insulin therapy is to efficiently control blood sugar levels by imitating the body's natural production of insulin. Insulin comes in four different formulation types: short-acting, intermediate-acting, long-acting, and rapid-acting. Insulin pumps or injections are two ways that insulin can be given.

Additional Therapies

To address type 2 diabetes and its consequences, additional treatment modalities may be employed, such as insulin therapy and oral medicine. These could consist of:

Bariatric Surgery: To achieve significant weight loss and increase insulin sensitivity, bariatric surgery may be considered for persons with extreme obesity and uncontrolled diabetes.

Continuous Glucose Monitoring (CGM) Systems: These devices offer real-time glucose monitoring, enabling users to keep tabs on their blood sugar levels and make educated choices regarding their food, exercise regimen, and dosage of medications.

Islet or Pancreas Cell Transplantation: To improve blood sugar regulation and restore insulin production, people with type 1 diabetes or some forms of type 2 diabetes may be candidates for islet or pancreas cell transplantation.

"The Type 2 Diabetes Solution" enables people with type 2 diabetes to collaborate with their healthcare professionals to create individualized treatment regimens that cater to their particular requirements and preferences by examining the range of medication and treatment alternatives that are available.

Chapter Four

Observation and Self-Management Techniques

Continuous monitoring of blood sugar levels and the application of self-care techniques to enhance general health and well-being are necessary for the effective management of type 2 diabetes. In "The Type 2 Diabetes Solution," we stress the need for self-care and self-monitoring methods for preserving ideal blood sugar regulation and averting problems.

Blood Sugar Tracking

For people with type 2 diabetes to control their blood sugar levels and make educated choices regarding their food, exercise regimen, and medication dosage, regular blood glucose monitoring is necessary. Typical techniques for blood glucose monitoring consist of:

Fingerstick testing is the process of measuring blood sugar levels from a little drop of blood collected by pricking the fingertip using a blood glucose meter.

Continuous Glucose Monitoring (CGM): CGM devices assess the amount of glucose in the interstitial fluid by implanting a small sensor beneath the skin to offer real-time glucose monitoring. Understanding glucose trends, patterns, and changes during the day and night can be greatly aided by CGM systems.

Flash Glucose Monitoring: Interstitial glucose levels are continuously measured by flash glucose monitoring devices using a tiny skin-attached sensor. Without doing a fingerstick test, users can receive glucose levels by using a reader device to scan the sensor.

Foot Hygiene

Type 2 diabetes raises the risk of foot issues by reducing blood flow to the feet and causing neuropathy (damage to the nerves) (peripheral arterial disease). It is possible to avoid foot ulcers, infections, and major consequences by taking good care of your feet. Important foot care techniques include:

Daily Inspection: Observe the foot every day for any signs of injury, such as cuts, blisters, redness, or swelling.

Appropriate Footwear: To prevent friction and harm to the feet, wear socks and shoes that fit well.

Frequent Foot Exams: Having a medical practitioner examine your feet frequently to evaluate your circulation, feelings, and overall health.

Dental and Eye Health

Diabetes mellitus type 2 can raise the risk of periodontal disease and diabetic retinopathy, two conditions that affect the eyes and gums. Regular dental and eye checkups are crucial for the early diagnosis and management of these disorders. Important suggestions consist of:

Annual Eye Exams: Getting a dilated eye exam every year from a qualified eye care specialist to check for complications with the eyes, such as diabetic retinopathy.

Frequent Dental Visits: Keeping your mouth healthy and preventing gum disease by scheduling routine cleanings and exams with a dentist.

People with type 2 diabetes can effectively manage their condition, lower their risk of complications, and enhance their overall quality of life by adopting self-care and monitoring methods into their daily routines. "The Type 2 Diabetes Solution" offers advice and materials to help readers put these crucial self-care techniques into practice.

Chapter Five

Establishing a Diabetes-Friendly Setting

In "The Type 2 Diabetes Solution," we stress how crucial it is to establish a welcoming atmosphere that encourages wholesome behaviors and makes managing diabetes easier. Simple adjustments made to the home, office, and social environments can help people with type 2 diabetes manage daily obstacles and maintain ideal blood sugar management.

Advice for Organising Meals and Grocery Shopping
Putting Up a Stockpile of Healthful Options: Stock the refrigerator and pantry with diabetes-friendly foods such as fruits, vegetables, whole grains, lean proteins, and healthy fats.

Reading Food Labels: Acquire the skill of reading food labels to spot packaged goods' hidden sugars, carbs, and unhealthy substances.

Meal Prepping: To minimize the temptation to choose unhealthy foods, prepare meals and snacks ahead of time and keep healthy options handy.

Techniques for Eating Out

Examining Menus in Advance: Look for diabetic-friendly options on restaurant menus online before going out to eat, and then adjust your meal plan accordingly.

Customizing Orders: Don't be afraid to ask for menu items to be changed, such as adding vegetables in place of starchy sides or asking for dressings and sauces to be served separately.

Portion control involves being aware of serving sizes and asking for a to-go box or splitting an entree to save half the meal for later.

Taking Care of Diabetes at Work

Stocking Nutritious Snacks: To prevent depending on vending machine selections, keep a supply of nutrient-dense snacks like nuts, seeds, yogurt, or chopped veggies at your desk.

Taking Regular Breaks: Throughout the workday, take brief breaks to stretch, move about, and check your blood sugar levels if necessary.

Interacting with Coworkers: Colleagues should be made aware of their diabetes care requirements, including the value of eating regular meals and snacks, and they should be taught what to do in the event of an emergency involving diabetes.

Getting Around in Social Situations

Bringing Food to Share: Make sure there are healthy options accessible at social gatherings by offering to bring a dish that is suitable for people with diabetes.

Preparing Ahead for Special Occasions: When attending parties or celebrations, schedule your meals and snacks in advance to prevent overindulging in high-calorie or sugary items.

Having a Support System: Be in the company of friends and family who are understanding of your dietary requirements and who support you in making healthy decisions.

People with type 2 diabetes can effectively manage their illness and lead satisfying, balanced lives by making their home, workplace, and social environments diabetes-friendly. "The Type 2 Diabetes Solution" offers helpful advice and methods for adjusting to different situations while putting general health and diabetes control first.

Chapter Six

Resources and Support Systems

According to "The Type 2 Diabetes Solution," having a solid support network and easy access to resources are critical for successfully treating type 2 diabetes. There are many ways for people with diabetes to get advice, encouragement, and useful help: from medical professionals and support groups to internet resources and smartphone apps.

The Value of Support Systems

Support on an Emotional Level: Managing a chronic illness such as type 2 diabetes can be emotionally taxing. During trying times, having a network of friends, family, and medical experts by your side can offer support, empathy, and a listening ear.

Practical Assistance: People with diabetes may find it easier to maintain healthy habits if they have support networks to help with chores like meal planning, grocery shopping, exercise regimens, and medication monitoring.

Accountability: By offering inspiration, encouragement, and tactful reminders to put their health first, being a part of a support network can help people stay accountable to their diabetes management goals.

Locating Support Groups and Educators for Diabetes

Diabetes Educators: Trained in diabetes management, certified diabetes educators (CDEs) are medical experts who can offer individualized guidance, counseling, and support to people with diabetes and their families. They can provide advice on how to manage medications, plan meals, check blood sugar, and make lifestyle changes.

Support Groups: Participating in a diabetes support group can help people meet people who are aware of the difficulties associated with having the disease. Support groups give a secure setting for people to talk about their experiences, trade advice, and techniques, and offer support and encouragement to one another.

Making Use of Mobile Apps and Online Resources

Websites for Education: There are a tonne of reliable websites and internet resources devoted to managing and educating people with diabetes. These websites provide information on diabetes and effective management techniques through articles, webinars, videos, and interactive tools.

Apps for mobile devices: A plethora of applications are available for managing diabetes on mobile devices, such as those that check blood sugar levels, keep an eye on food intake, log physical activity, schedule medicine reminders, and establish connections with medical professionals. People with diabetes can benefit from these apps by staying motivated, organized, and involved in their care.

People with type 2 diabetes can acquire the information, self-assurance, and practical skills necessary to effectively manage their condition and lead fulfilling lives with diabetes by leveraging available resources and connecting with support networks. To empower readers on their diabetes journey, "The Type 2 Diabetes

Solution" offers advice on where to
look for and how to use resources and
support networks.

Chapter Seven

Overcoming Obstacles and Maintaining Motivation

We agree in "The Type 2 Diabetes Solution" that managing type 2 diabetes can involve several problems, including changing one's lifestyle and adhering to drug regimens. But with the correct approaches and frame of mind, people can get past these challenges and continue to be inspired to put their health and well-being first.

Handling Relapses and Setbacks

Self-Compassion: It's critical to cultivate self-compassion and accept that obstacles are a typical aspect of managing diabetes. Consider taking what you can from the event and pressing forward with newfound vigor rather than obsessing over past mistakes.

Finding Triggers: Consider the elements that might have led to the failure, such as stress, emotional eating, or a deficiency of support. People can create proactive ways to deal with these issues by identifying triggers.

Seeking Support: In trying times, rely on your network of friends, family, medical professionals, and support organizations. Talking to people about your difficulties can help you gain important perspective, support, and useful guidance.

Establishing Objectives and Monitoring Development

Setting Achievable and Realistic Goals: Make sure your goals are time-bound, relevant, measurable, specified, and reachable (SMART). To keep the momentum going and recognize minor victories along the way, break down more ambitious objectives into more doable chunks.

Monitoring Your Progress: Use a notebook, smartphone app, wearable gadget, or other appropriate tool to keep tabs on your blood sugar levels, medication compliance, eating habits, physical activity, and other pertinent data. Tracking development can inspire behavior change, reveal trends, and offer insightful information.

Rewarding Yourself: Celebrate your progress and accomplishments to keep yourself inspired. Simple pleasures like watching a movie, taking a soothing bath, or spending time with close friends and family can serve as rewards.

Honouring Achievers and Significant Occasions

Acknowledging Successes: No matter how minor, acknowledge and appreciate your accomplishments. Whether it's hitting a blood sugar goal, adhering to a nutritious diet, or hitting a personal fitness benchmark, celebrate your successes and recognize the work that went into them.

Sharing Success Stories: Talk about your achievements with members of the diabetes community or in your support system. Your stories can encourage and uplift those going through comparable difficulties, creating a bond and a sense of community.

Examining Your Progress: Consider the distance you've traveled since you began managing your diabetes. Acknowledge the improvements you've made and the effects they've had on your well-being.

People with type 2 diabetes can overcome obstacles and maintain motivation to lead healthier, more rewarding lives by taking a proactive mentality, setting realistic objectives, getting help when required, and celebrating small victories along the way. "The Type 2 Diabetes Solution" offers readers support and techniques to help them remain resolute and committed to their diabetes care objectives.

Chapter Eight

Particular Aspects and Difficulties

We discuss special considerations and potential difficulties that people with type 2 diabetes may experience in "The Type 2 Diabetes Solution." It is vital to comprehend these characteristics to manage the condition efficiently and lower the likelihood of complications.

Heart health and diabetes

Elevated Risk of Cardiovascular Diseases: People with type 2 diabetes are more likely to experience heart attacks, strokes, and peripheral artery disease. Prioritizing heart health through dietary changes, medication administration, and routine monitoring of cardiovascular risk variables like blood pressure, cholesterol, and blood sugar regulation is essential.

Cardiac Screening: To evaluate heart function and identify early indicators of cardiovascular disease, routine cardiac screenings, such as electrocardiograms (ECGs), echocardiograms, and stress tests, may be advised for people with diabetes.

Kidney disease and diabetes

Diabetic Nephropathy: Also known as kidney disease, diabetic nephropathy is a frequent side effect of type 2 diabetes that, if uncontrolled, can result in kidney failure. Regular blood and urine testing to monitor kidney function is crucial for early detection and treatment.

Blood Pressure Control: To stop or slow the development of diabetic kidney disease, blood pressure management is essential. A low-sodium diet, frequent exercise, and medication management are examples of lifestyle changes that can lower blood pressure and safeguard renal function.

Diabetes and Eye Conditions

Diabetic Retinopathy: One of the main causes of blindness and vision loss in people with type 2 diabetes is diabetic retinopathy. Appropriate eye examinations by an optometrist or ophthalmologist are necessary for diabetic retinopathy early diagnosis and therapy.

Blood Sugar Control: Preventing or postponing the development and progression of diabetic retinopathy requires strict blood sugar management. Maintaining control over other controllable risk factors, such as cholesterol and blood pressure, can also assist in safeguarding eye health.

Pregnancy and Diabetes

Diabetes that develops during pregnancy is known as gestational diabetes, and it can raise the mother's and the unborn child's risk of complications. It is imperative to manage gestational diabetes appropriately with food, exercise, and medication if needed to ensure a safe pregnancy and delivery.

Preconception Counselling: To improve blood sugar control and lower the risk of pregnancy-related problems, women with type 2 diabetes who intend to get pregnant should undergo preconception counseling.

People with type 2 diabetes can take proactive measures to safeguard their health, avoid complications, and improve their results by attending to these unique considerations and issues related to the disease. "The Type 2 Diabetes Solution" offers advice and tools to assist readers in overcoming these obstacles and successfully managing their disease.

Chapter Nine

Considering the Future

We examine the exciting new directions and prospects for diabetes care and treatment in "The Type 2 Diabetes Solution." For those with type 2 diabetes, improvements in science, technology, and healthcare delivery provide hope for better results and a higher standard of living.

Progress in the Study of Diabetes

Precision medicine: Scientists are trying to create individualized treatment plans based on a person's genetic composition, lifestyle choices, and illness features. The ultimate goal of precision medicine is to improve treatment outcomes and efficacy by customising diabetes management strategies to each individual's needs. Researchers are looking into ways to repair or regenerate the beta cells in the pancreas that produce insulin; this could potentially help people with type 2 diabetes regain normal insulin activity over the long term.

Prospective Technologies and Interventions

Systems for Continuous Glucose Monitoring (CGM): Continuous glucose monitoring systems are still developing due to improvements in data analytic capabilities, wearability, and sensor accuracy. More accuracy, ease, and integration with other diabetes management technologies could be provided by future CGM systems.

Closed-Loop Systems: Also referred to as artificial pancreas systems, closed-loop systems use automated insulin delivery in conjunction with continuous glucose monitoring to control blood sugar levels in real-time. These technologies have the potential to lessen the burden of managing type 2 diabetes on those with the disease while simultaneously enhancing glycemic control.

Living Well with Diabetes: Inspiring and Optimistic Narratives

Patient Empowerment and Advocacy: Individuals with diabetes are progressively taking on the role of self and community advocates, bringing attention to issues, pushing for legislative reforms, and encouraging accessibility to resources and care for the disease.

Living a Fulfilling Life Despite Diabetes: Despite the difficulties associated with managing their condition, many people with type 2 diabetes are reaching their goals and leading fulfilling lives. These people encourage others to take charge of their health and achieve their goals by sharing their tales of resiliency, tenacity, and accomplishment.

It's critical to maintain optimism and initiative as we consider new developments in diabetes care, push for better treatment, and encourage one another on the path to greater health and well-being. "The Type 2 Diabetes Solution" exhorts readers to maintain an informed, involved, and optimistic outlook toward their prospects for a better future while managing diabetes.